Sprint Count Calories Cookbook for Fledglings

Healthy lifestyle to lower blood pressure

Thomas Grey

Table of contents

Introduction

The Sprint Count Calories Cookbook for Beginners is a comprehensive guide designed to help beginners navigate the world of calorie counting and adopt a healthier lifestyle. Created specifically for those new to calorie counting, this cookbook offers valuable insights, delicious recipes, and practical tips aimed at improving your health and well-being.

Calorie counting is a proven method for weight management, improved nutrition, and achieving fitness goals. Understanding the importance of calorie intake and making informed choices about the foods you consume can have a significant impact on your overall health and vitality. With this cookbook, beginners can learn the basics of calorie counting and discover a variety of delicious recipes that are nutritious and filling.

The cookbook features a variety of recipes covering different food categories such as breakfast, lunch, dinner, snacks, and desserts.

Each recipe is carefully crafted to provide detailed nutritional information, with a specific focus on calories, to help individuals effectively monitor their daily intake. From simple and easy meals to elaborate dishes, this cookbook offers a variety of options for different tastes and dietary preferences.

In addition to the recipe book, the cookbook also includes guidance on meal planning, portion control, how to read food labels, and common mistakes to avoid when counting calories.

It also addresses specific health issues such as lowering blood pressure and reducing salt intake, and provides specific meal plans and recipes to reach those goals. Whether you're looking to lose a few pounds, improve your overall health, or simply want to understand more about the foods you're eating, the Sprint Count Calories Cookbook for Chicks is an invaluable resource.

It provides beginners with the knowledge and tools they need to confidently embark on their calorie-counting journey, helping them make informed decisions and reach their health and wellness goals. Grab your apron, get ready to explore a world of delicious and nutritious recipes, and take the first step towards a healthier, happier person.

Chapter 1

The Importance of Counting Calories

In the modern world, where healthy food options are readily available and portion sizes are dramatically increased, calorie counting has become an essential tool for those who want to maintain healthy weight management and improve their overall health. By understanding and tracking the number of calories consumed each day, beginners can take control of their nutrition and make informed choices that align with their health and fitness goals. "The Sprint Beginner Calorie Cookbook" recognizes the importance of counting calories and aims to guide those new to the process.

Calorie counting involves tracking the energy content of foods and beverages consumed. It provides a quantitative measurement of the amount of fuel the body is receiving. This information is important because body weight is determined by the balance between calories taken in and calories burned. When calorie intake exceeds energy expenditure, the excess calories are stored as fat, leading to weight gain over time. On the other hand, expending less calories than your body needs can lead to weight misfortune.

By counting calories, individuals better understand their energy intake and can adjust accordingly. This allows them to identify areas where their diet may be in excess or lacking in essential nutrients. Counting calories isn't just about limiting, it's about making informed choices and achieving balance. It helps individuals become aware of their eating habits, portion sizes, and nutritional value of the foods they eat.

The "Sprint Calorie Cookbook for Toddlers" offers a wide range of delicious and nutritious recipes with detailed calorie information. This allows beginners to make informed decisions about the foods they like and ensure they are within the desired calorie range.

By incorporating these recipes into their daily meal plans, individuals can create balanced and satisfying meals while still meeting their calorie goals. In addition to weight management, counting calories can also benefit people with specific health concerns, such as those aiming to lower blood pressure or reduce sodium intake. By tracking calories, individuals can tailor their diets to support these goals, ultimately leading to better overall health.

It's important to note that calorie counting should be done with a balanced mindset. This is not about deprivation or rigid rules but about sustainable lifestyle changes. The Sprint Count Calories Cookbook for beginners emphasizes the importance of listening to your body, practicing portion control, and eating a variety of nutrient-dense foods to support your overall health and wellness.

In summary, calorie counting is a powerful tool that enables individuals to manage their diet, make informed decisions, and achieve their health and fitness goals. The Sprint Calorie Counting Cookbook for Beginners serves as a comprehensive beginner's guide with knowledge, recipes, and strategies to successfully complete your calorie-counting journey and begin your journey to a healthier and happier lifestyle.

Benefits of meal preparation

Meal prep has become more popular in recent years and with good reason. The Sprint Count Calories Cookbook for Fldglings recognizes the many benefits of meal prep, especially for those new to calorie counting and looking to improve their diet and overall health.

Here are some of the key benefits of incorporating meal prep into your routine.

Time efficiency

One of the main benefits of meal prep is that it saves you time. Setting aside a specific amount of time each week for meal planning, shopping, and preparation can streamline the cooking process. That means less time in the kitchen and more ready-to-eat meals on busy weekdays. Preparing meals gives you valuable time for other activities, reduces stress, and ensures healthy eating.

Part control

Once the dinner preparations are complete, there is an opportunity to distribute the dinner in progress. This allows you to control portion sizes and consume just the right amount of calories to reach your goals. Having pre-portioned meals on hand can help you avoid the temptation to overeat or resort to unhealthy convenience foods. Managing meal size is an important aspect of calorie counting, and meal preparation promotes this habit.

Nutritional balance

Meal preparation promotes a balanced and nutritious diet. By planning and preparing your meals in advance, you can include a variety of fruits, vegetables, lean proteins, whole grains, and healthy fats in every meal. This will help you meet your nutritional needs and ensure you are eating a balanced diet. Having ready-made meals available means you're less likely to resort to unhealthy foods when you're hungry.

Fetched Investment funds

Supper prepping can moreover lead to money-related investment funds. By arranging your dinners in development and obtaining fixings in bulk, you'll be able to take advantage of rebates and diminish nourishment squandering. Moreover, by bringing pre-prepared dinners with you to work or school, you'll maintain a strategic distance from exorbitant takeout or eatery dinners. Over time, these investment funds can make feast prepping a budget-friendly alternative.

Diminished Push

The comfort and organization that come with feast prepping can essentially diminish push levels. Knowing that you simply have solid and fulfilling suppers prepared to enjoy eliminates the requirement for last-minute choices or hurried cooking. By having an arrangement in put and dinners arranged, you'll be able to approach your week with a sense of calm and certainty, knowing that your nourishment is taken care of.

Moved forward with Dietary Compliance

For people with particular dietary necessities or well-being objectives, dinner prepping can be especially useful. Whether you're taking after a calorie-controlled eat less, a low-sodium arrangement, or any other specialized eating approach, dinner prepping permits you to follow your dietary needs with ease. Having dinners arranged in progress expels the mystery and allurements, making a difference in your remaining on track and keeping up dietary compliance.

Consolidating feast prepping into your schedule can be a game-changer when it comes to achieving your well-being and wellness objectives. The Sprint Number Calories Cookbook for Youth provides guidance on feast preparation techniques and offers recipes suitable for on-the-fly planning. By grasping the hone of dinner prepping, you'll appreciate the comfort, reserve funds, and dietary benefits that it brings, eventually supporting your travel towards a more beneficial and more balanced lifestyle.

Understanding Sodium and Its Effect on Well-being

Sodium is a basic mineral that plays a crucial part in the body's functioning. However, over-the-top sodium admissions can have critical suggestions for by and large well-being. The "Sprint Check Calories Cookbook for Juveniles" recognizes the significance of understanding sodium and its effect on well-being, especially for people who are modern to checking calories and looking to make strides in their well-being.

Here is an outline of sodium and its impacts

Sodium and Fluid Adjustment

Sodium makes a difference by direct liquid adjustment within the body by controlling the development of water over cell films. Satisfactory sodium admissions are vital for keeping up appropriate hydration and guaranteeing the ideal working of cells, tissues, and organs. Be that as it may, over-the-top sodium utilization can disturb this adjustment, driving fluid retention and possibly contributing to conditions like tall blood weight.

Sodium and Blood Weight

All sodium intake is unequivocally related to expanded blood weight levels. When sodium levels within the body rise, it draws in water, driving liquid maintenance and an increment in blood volume. This, in turn, puts a more prominent strain on the heart and blood vessels, lifting blood weight. Delayed tall blood weight can increment the chance of heart disease, stroke, and other cardiovascular complications.

Sodium and Kidney Work

The kidneys play a noteworthy portion in controlling sodium levels inside the body. They offer assistance with channel overabundance of sodium and keep up a sound adjustment. Be that as it may, a reliably tall sodium slim down can put a strain on the kidneys, affecting their capacity to operate ideally. Over time, this will lead to impaired kidney work and increases the hazard of kidney illness

Sodium and Bone Health

Sodium is necessary for many bodily functions, but excessive sodium intake can adversely affect bone health. High sodium levels increase urinary excretion of calcium, which can lead to calcium deficiency and loss of bone density. This can increase the risk of osteoporosis and fractures.

Sodium and general health

In addition to the specific health problems mentioned above, excessive sodium intake is also associated with other health problems, such as an increased risk of stomach cancer, fluid retention, and bloating.

Reducing your sodium intake and maintaining a balanced diet will contribute to your overall health and help prevent these health complications. To effectively manage your sodium intake, it is important to be aware of hidden sources of sodium in your diet. Processed and packaged foods such as canned soups, snack foods, sauces, and condiments often contain large amounts of sodium.

By reading food labels and choosing low-sodium alternatives, you can significantly reduce your sodium consumption. The Sprint Count Calories Cookbook for chicks includes recipes and tips for reducing salt in their diets while maintaining flavor and nutritional value.

By understanding sodium and its effects on health, individuals can make informed dietary choices and implement strategies to reduce sodium intake. Counting calories and monitoring sodium levels can help you achieve a healthier balance and promote overall wellness.

The Sprint Count Calories Cookbook for Fldglings supports an individual's mindful eating journey, empowering them to make choices that contribute to their long-term health and vitality.

Chapter 2

Start Counting Calories

What are calories?

A calorie is a unit of energy. In the context of nutrition, it refers to the amount of energy you get when you consume food or drink. Calories are essential for the body's daily activities, including physical activity, metabolic processes, and maintaining organ function.

Calorie counting basics

Calorie counting is an essential practice for anyone looking to control their weight, improve their diet, or achieve specific health and fitness goals.

Understanding the basics of calorie counting can give beginners valuable insight into their eating habits and help them make informed decisions about the foods they eat.

The Sprint Counting Calorie Cookbook for Chicks is intended to provide a clear understanding of this process and give individuals control over their diet.

The important basics of calorie counting are:

Calories in and out

Calorie intake is the number of calories consumed through food and drink. Calorie expenditure refers to the number of calories expended through physical activity and metabolic processes. To control your weight, it's important to keep a balance between your calorie intake and your calorie expenditure. Eating more calories than your body needs will make you gain weight while eating fewer calories will make you lose weight.

Read the food label

The food name provides important information about the nutritional content of the food in the bundle. When calculating calories, keep in mind the serving size and the number of calories per serving. This allows you to accurately track your calorie intake. Food labels also provide information about other nutrients such as fats, carbohydrates, proteins, and fiber that are important in a balanced diet.

Calorie intake tracking

To effectively calculate calories, it helps you track your daily food and drink consumption. This can be done in several ways, such as keeping a food journal, using mobile apps and online tools, or relying on printed resources. A sprint counting calorie cookbook for chicks may provide a tracking sheet or recommend specific resources to help with this process.

Calorie database and references

When counting calories, it's helpful to have access to a comprehensive calorie database or reference book. These resources provide information on the caloric content of various foods and beverages, including fresh produce, common ingredients, and processed foods. A sprint counting calorie cookbook for chicks may include an informative section or suggest authoritative sources for accurate calorie information.

Accuracy and Consistency

Accurate and consistent calorie counting is critical to getting the results you want. Watch your portions, measure your ingredients accurately, and keep track of everything you eat. By continuously tracking your calorie intake, you can identify patterns, make adjustments as needed, and stay accountable.

By mastering the basics of calorie counting, individuals can make informed decisions about their eating habits, portions, and total calorie intake. The Sprint Count Calories Cookbook for Beginners serves as a valuable resource providing helpful steps, recipes, and strategies for beginning calorie counters. Remember, counting calories is not about restricting your calorie intake, it's about creating a healthy balance that helps you stay healthy and reach your health and fitness goals.

Determine your calorie needs

Understanding your personal calorie needs is an important step in effectively counting calories and achieving your health and fitness goals. The Sprint Count Calories Cookbook for Fledglings recognizes the importance of this process and provides guidance to help beginners determine exactly how many calories they need. The main factors to consider when determining your calorie needs are:

Basal Metabolic Rate (BMR)

Basal metabolic rate (BMR) refers to the number of calories your body needs to maintain basic physiological functions at rest. It is responsible for processes such as respiration, blood circulation, cell production, and body temperature maintenance. Several factors affect her BMR, including age, gender, weight, and height. Calculating your BMR gives you a basis for estimating your daily calorie needs.

Physical activity level

Your level of physical activity plays an important role in determining your calorie needs. Physical activity includes not only systematic exercise but also daily activities such as walking, cleaning, and gardening. A sedentary lifestyle requires fewer calories than a very active lifestyle. Consider your activity level when estimating how many calories you need to maintain or reach your goal.

The goal

Your health and fitness goals affect your calorie needs. On the off chance that your objective is weight misfortune, you wish a calorie shortfall. This means that you take in fewer calories than your body uses. If your goal is to maintain weight or build muscle, your caloric intake should match or slightly exceed your energy expenditure. Setting clear goals can help you adjust your calorie intake accordingly.

Body composition

Body composition, such as muscle mass and body fat percentage, affects how many calories you need. Muscle tissue is metabolically active and requires more calories to maintain. More muscle mass increases your BMR and therefore your calorie needs. In general, people with more muscle mass need more calories than people with more body fat.

Talk to an expert

Online calculators and formulas can give you an estimate, but we recommend consulting a registered dietitian or healthcare professional to determine your exact calorie needs.

They will consider your unique situation, assess your health and provide personalized recommendations based on your goals. It's important to remember that determining calorie needs is not an exact science and varies from person to person. Experimentation and confidence are essential. Monitor your progress, adjust your calorie intake as needed, and pay attention to your body's hunger and satiety signals.

The Sprint Count Calorie Cookbook for Chicks may contain resources, references, or recommendations for calculating calorie needs.

It is important to use the calorie estimate as a starting point and adjust it based on individual reactions and body feedback.

By accurately grasping and determining your calorie needs, you can set the appropriate calorie intake according to your goals. This knowledge allows you to make informed decisions about portion sizes, meal planning, and balanced meals.

The Sprint Count Calories Cookbook for Beginners supports a beginner's calorie counting journey by providing tools and strategies to effectively identify and meet individual calorie needs.

Following and Observing Caloric Admissions
Following and checking your caloric admissions may be a significant angle of tallying calories and accomplishing your well-being and wellness objectives. By keeping a record of the nourishments and refreshments you devour, you

pick up profitable knowledge about your dietary propensities and can make educated choices to bolster your objectives. The "Sprint Number Calories Cookbook for Juveniles" recognizes the significance of following and offers direction on successfully monitoring caloric intake.

Here are a couple of key centers to consider:

Select a Following Strategy
Select the following strategy that suits your inclinations and way of life. There are different alternatives accessible, counting conventional pen-and-paper nourishment diaries, portable apps, online apparatuses, or printable layouts. The critical thing is to discover a strategy that's convenient and simple for you to utilize reliably.

Track Everything You Expend
To induce a precise picture of your caloric admissions, it's critical to track everything you eat and drink. This incorporates suppers, snacks, refreshments, condiments, and cooking oils. Pay consideration to parcel sizes and utilize

measuring apparatuses when essential to guarantee precision.

Examined and Record Nourishment Names
When following calories, read and record the dietary data from nourishment names. Pay consideration to serving sizes and the number of calories per serving. In the event that you're employing a following app or online device, numerous of them have a database of pre-entered nourishment things with their dietary data, making it simpler to track your admissions precisely.

Be Careful of Cooking Strategies
Consider the cooking strategies utilized and any included fixings that contribute to the caloric substance of your dinners. This incorporates oils, sauces, dressings, and seasonings. When following, account for these increases to guarantee a precise representation of your general caloric admissions.

Degree Fixings

When cooking at domestic, use measuring glasses, spoons, or a nourishment scale to degree fixings. This makes a difference guarantee precision in following the calories of homemade dinners and formulas. It's particularly imperative for calorie-dense fixings like oils, nuts, and grains.

Feasting Out and Social Settings

When eating out or going to social occasions, evaluating calories can be more challenging. Be that as it may, numerous eateries and fast-food chains presently give dietary data for their menus things. Utilize online resources or portable apps to seek calorie data when eating out. In case particular information isn't accessible, make your best estimation based on comparable nourishments or fixings.

Remain Steady and Responsible

Consistency is key when following caloric admissions. Make it a propensity to record your nourishment and refreshment consumption regularly. This hone makes a difference and increases self-awareness and holds you responsible for your choices. Over time, you'll create a distant better; a much better; a higher; a stronger; and improved stronger understanding of parcel sizes and the caloric substance of distinctive nourishments.

Screen Advance and Alter

Following your caloric intake permits you to screen your advance toward your objectives. Routinely audit your records and evaluate how your body responds to the calories expended. In the event that is vital, make alterations to your caloric admissions based on your advance and counsel a healthcare proficient or registered dietitian for personalized direction.

The "Sprint Number Calories Cookbook for Juveniles" may give the following sheets or suggest particular assets to help you in following and checking your caloric admissions viably. By keeping up a reliable following, you'll be able to pick up experiences into your eating habits, identify ranges for enhancement, and make educated choices to back your by and large well-being.

Tips for Successful Calorie Counting

Calorie counting can be a powerful strategy for weight management, improved nutrition, and achieving specific health goals. To ensure a successful calorie-counting journey, the "Sprint Count Calories Cookbook for Fledglings" offers helpful tips and guides to make the process easier and more effective.

Here are some key tips for successful calorie counting.

Set realistic goals

First, set realistic and achievable goals. Whether your goals are weight loss, weight maintenance, or muscle gain, make sure your goals are specific, measurable, achievable, relevant, and time-bound (SMART). please. Setting realistic goals keeps you motivated and ensures continuous progress.

For Yourself

Take the time to learn about the nutrition, portion sizes, and calorie content of different foods. Understanding the nutritional components of foods and how they contribute to total caloric intake allows you to make informed choices and plan a balanced diet.

Use trusted resources

Get accurate information about the calorie content of foods with trusted resources like trusted calorie databases, nutrition labels, and tracking apps. The Sprint Count Calories Cookbook for Beginners may recommend specific resources to help you track and count calories effectively.

Measure out

Invest in measuring cups, spoons, and food scales to accurately measure portions. Estimating portions can lead to inaccurate calorie calculations. By measuring your food, you can get a more accurate picture of your calorie consumption.

Watch out for hidden calories

Pay attention to hidden calorie sources, especially in condiments, sauces, dressings, and beverages. These items can contribute a significant portion of your daily caloric intake. Choose low-calorie or low-fat alternatives whenever possible, or consider making a homemade version.

Meal planning and preparation

Meal planning and preparation are key to successful calorie counting. Take the time to plan your meals in advance, considering the calories and nutritional value of each dish. The Sprint Count Calories Cookbook for chicks includes meal plans, recipes, and instructions for preparing balanced,
calorie-controlled meals.

Be consistent

Consistency is the key to successful calorie counting. Get in the habit of monitoring your calories every day, including weekends and holidays. Being consistent helps you take responsibility and have a clearer picture of your overall calorie intake.

Practice partial control

Portion control is important when counting calories. Be mindful of portion sizes and pay attention to your body's hunger and nutritional needs. Avoid overeating and be mindful of portions, especially when eating out or eating prepackaged meals.

Find support

Consider finding support systems and accountability partners who share similar goals and interests. Sometimes it helps to have someone with whom you can share your progress, challenges, and successes. Additionally, personalized guidance and support are provided with advice from a certified dietician or health professional.

Enjoy your meal flexibly

Remember, calorie counting is a tool that supports health and well-being. Be flexible and plan occasional rewards and special occasions. Enjoy the foods you love and try to eat a balanced and sustainable diet.

Practicing these tips will improve your calorie-counting experience and increase your chances of reaching your health and fitness goals.

The Sprint Count Calories Cookbook for Beginners is designed to help calorie-counting beginners by providing practical tips, delicious recipes, and how-to guides to develop a healthy, mindful approach to eating.

Chapter 3

Sprint Low-Sodium Supper Formulas

Herb-Roasted Chicken with Steamed Vegetables

This formula for herb-roasted chicken with steamed vegetables may be a nutritious and flavorful dinner that can be delighted in as a portion of an adjusted count of calories. It combines delicate and delicious chicken with a mixture of colorful vegetables, prepared with fragrant herbs. The "Sprint Check Calories Cookbook for Juveniles" presents this tasty formula as an illustration of a sound and calorie-conscious dish.

Here's how to plan herb-roasted chicken with steamed vegetables:

Fixings
4 boneless, skinless chicken breasts
2 tablespoons olive oil
1 tablespoon new lemon juice
1 teaspoon dried rosemary
1 teaspoon dried thyme
1 teaspoon dried oregano
1/2 teaspoon garlic powder
Salt and pepper to taste
2 mugs blended vegetables such as carrots, broccoli, and chime peppers, cut into bite-sized pieces

Informational

Preheat your broiler to 400°F (200°C).
In a little bowl, combine the olive oil, lemon juice, dried rosemary, dried thyme, dried oregano, garlic powder, salt, and pepper. Blend well to make a marinade.

Put the chicken breasts in a shallow dish and pour the marinade on top. Make beyond any doubt the chicken is equitably coated. Permit it to marinate for at least 15 minutes to upgrade the flavors.

Whereas the chicken is marinating, get ready the vegetables. Wash and cut them into bite-sized pieces. You'll select any combination of vegetables you lean toward or have on hand.

Put water in a pot and bring it to a bubble. Put a steamer wicker container on the top of the pot, guaranteeing that it doesn't touch the water. Include the vegetables in the steamer wicker container, cover with a top, and steam for approximately 5-7 minutes, or until they are tender-crisp. Take care not to overcook the vegetables to hold their supplements and dynamic colors.

Whereas the vegetables are steaming, warm a non-stick skillet over medium-high heat. Once hot, include the marinated chicken breasts in the skillet. Burn each side for almost 2-3 minutes, or until they develop a golden-brown hull.

Put the fricasseed chicken breast in a casserole dish and put it on the preheated stove. Cook for roughly 15-20 minutes, or until the chicken comes to an inside temperature of 165°F (74°C) and is cooked through. The cooking time may move depending on the thickness of the chicken breasts.

Once the chicken is cooked, clear it from the broiler and let it rest for a few minutes, sometime recently cutting.

Serve the herb-roasted chicken with the steamed vegetable on the side. You'll be able to decorate with extra new herbs in case you want.

This herb-roasted chicken with steamed vegetables formula gives an adjusted combination of incline protein from the chicken and a grouping of vitamins, minerals, and dietary fiber from the vegetables. It may be a flexible dish that can be delighted in for lunch or supper, and it can be effectively customized by including your favorite herbs or flavors.
 Remember to adjust portions based on your individual calorie needs and goals. The Sprint Count Calories Cookbook for Beginners provides nutritional information and presentation suggestions to help beginners effectively monitor their calorie intake while enjoying these delicious and healthy meals.

Grilled fish tacos with fresh salsa
Grilled Fish Tacos with Fresh Salsa combine the flavors of tender grilled fish, rich salsa, and warm tortillas in a delicious and healthy dish.

This recipe from the Sprint Count Calories Cookbook for Fledglings is a delicious way to enjoy a light, nutritious meal.

To make grilled fish tacos with fresh salsa:

Material For fish
1 pound of fillet of white fish, such as tilapia, cod, or snapper. 1 tablespoon olive oil
1 teaspoon chili powder
1/2 teaspoon cumin
1/2 teaspoon paprika
salt and pepper to taste

For fresh salsa
1 cup diced tomatoes
1/2 cup chopped red onion
1/4 cup chopped fresh coriander
1 jalapeno pepper, seeded and finely chopped (for seasoning).
1 tablespoon fresh lime juice
taste with salt

To provide
8 small corn tortillas
sliced lime

Optional toppings
grated lettuce, sliced avocado, Greek yogurt, or
sour cream

Procedure
Preheat the grill to medium-high heat.
Alternatively, you can use a grill pan or stovetop
pan.

Mix olive oil, chili powder, cumin, paprika, salt,
and pepper in a small bowl. Stir well to create a
spice blend. Pat the fish fillets dry with a paper
towel and brush both sides with the spice
mixture.

Place the fish fillet on a preheated grill and grill
for about 3 to 4 minutes per side or until the fish
is opaque and can be shredded easily with a fork.
Baking time may vary depending on fillet
thickness.

While the fish is grilling, prepare the fresh salsa. In a medium bowl, combine diced tomatoes, red onion, cilantro, jalapeno peppers (if using), lime juice, and salt. Mix well to combine all flavors. Alter the flavors agreeing to your taste inclinations.

Heat corn tortillas on a grill or stovetop until soft and pliable. This process improves the flavor and makes it easier to fold.

Once the fish is cooked, remove it from the grill and let it sit for a few minutes. Then cut the fish into small pieces with a fork.

Assemble the grilled fish tacos by placing a generous amount of fish flakes on top of each heated tortilla. Top with a spoonful of fresh salsa and your choice of shredded lettuce, sliced avocado, or Greek yogurt.

Serve the grilled fish tacos immediately with a lime wedge to squeeze over the tacos. Enjoy it while it's fresh and flavorful. Grilled Fish Tacos with Fresh Salsa offer a delicious combination of flavors and textures, with smoky, tender fish complemented by a lively, tangy salsa.

The Sprint Count Calories Cookbook for Beginners provides serving suggestions and nutritional information to help beginners effectively monitor their calorie intake while enjoying this delicious and healthy meal.

Adjust amounts of spices, toppings, and tortilla options to suit your taste and dietary needs. Whether you're cooking a casual weeknight dinner or hosting a gathering, these grilled fish tacos are sure to impress and satisfy your taste buds while serving a nutritious meal.

Lemon Garlic Shrimp Stir-Fry

Lemon garlic shrimp stir-fry could be a fast, flavorful, and nutritious dish that exhibits the fragile and juicy flavors of shrimp combined with dynamic vegetables and fragrant seasonings. This formula, included within the "Sprint Check Calories Cookbook for

Juveniles," offers a tasty choice for a light and fulfilling supper.

Here's how to plan lemon garlic shrimp stir-fry:

Fixings
1 pound huge shrimp, peeled and deveined
2 tablespoons olive oil
4 garlic cloves, minced
1 teaspoon ground lemon get-up-and-go
2 tablespoons new lemon juice
1 tablespoon low-sodium soy sauce
1 tablespoon nectar
1 teaspoon cornstarch
Salt and pepper to taste
2 mugs blended vegetables such as chime peppers, snap peas, and carrots, daintily cut
1 teaspoon of sesame oil discretionary, for included flavor
2 green onions, cut for decoration.
Cooked rice or noodles for serving

Enlightening

In a little bowl, whisk together the minced garlic, lemon zest, lemon juice, soy sauce, nectar, cornstarch, salt, and pepper to form the sauce. Set aside. Warm the olive oil in a broad skillet or wok over medium-high heat.

Incorporate the shrimp into the skillet and cook for 2-3 minutes per side, until they turn pink and dull. Look out not to overcook the shrimp, as they can get rubbery. Oust the cooked shrimp from the skillet and set aside.

Within the same skillet, include the cut blended vegetables. Stir-fry for around 3-4 minutes, or until they are tender-crisp. The cooking time may alter depending on the thickness of the vegetables. Return the boiled shrimp to the pot along with the vegetables.

Pour the arranged sauce over the shrimp and vegetables. Blend well to coat everything equally. Cook for an extra 1-2 minutes, or until the sauce thickens marginally.

Discretionary

Sprinkle the sesame oil over the stir-fry and hurl to combine. Sesame oil includes a nutty flavor.

Expel the skillet from warm and embellish with cut green onions.

Serve the lemon garlic shrimp stir-fried hot cooked rice or noodles. The light and reviving flavors of the lemon and garlic will complement the juicy shrimp and dynamic vegetables.

This lemon garlic shrimp stir-fry could be a flexible dish that can be customized to suit your inclinations. Feel free to include or substitute vegetables based on what you have on hand. The "Sprint Number Calories Cookbook for Juveniles" may provide serving proposals and nutritional data to help fledglings in following their caloric admissions successfully whereas getting a charge out of this flavorful and wholesome dinner.

Keep in mind to alter the parcel sizes of rice or noodles agreeing to your personal caloric needs and objectives. With its bright flavors and adjusted combination of protein and vegetables, this stir-fry may be a scrumptious and nutritious choice for a fast and satisfying meal.

Prepared Salmon with Dill and Asparagus
Prepared salmon with dill and asparagus may be a healthy and flavorful dish that highlights the common lavishness of salmon combined with the new flavors of dill and delicate asparagus. This formula, highlighted within the "Sprint Check Calories Cookbook for Juveniles," offers a straightforward but delightful choice for a nutritious supper.

To make baked salmon with dill and asparagus:

Material
4 salmon fillets, about 6 ounces each
1 bunch asparagus, trimmed
2 tablespoons olive oil

2 tablespoons fresh lemon juice
2 tablespoons freshly chopped dill
salt and pepper to taste
lemon wedges for serving

Procedure

Preheat the oven to 400°F (200°C). Line a baking sheet with parchment paper or foil for easy cleaning.

Place the salmon fillets skin side down on the prepared baking sheet. Arrange the sliced asparagus next to the salmon.

In a small bowl, combine olive oil, lemon juice, chopped dill, salt, and pepper. Sprinkle this mixture evenly over the salmon and asparagus, making sure they are well coated.

Using your hands or a brush, gently rub the marinade into the salmon fillet and asparagus spears to evenly season.

Place the baking sheet in a preheated oven and bake for about 12 to 15 minutes or until the salmon is tender and easy to cut with a fork. Baking time may vary depending on the thickness of the salmon fillet.

After cooking, evacuate the heating sheet from the broiler. Let the salmon rest for a few minutes before eating.

Serve the grilled salmon with dill and asparagus, plus fresh dill and lemon wedges to squeeze over the salmon. Dill and lemon give the dish a refreshing aroma.

Baked salmon with dill and asparagus is a nutritious and filling meal, rich in omega-3 fatty acids from salmon and various vitamins and minerals from asparagus. Sprint Count Calories Cookbook for Beginners provides serving suggestions and nutritional information to help beginners effectively monitor their calorie intake while enjoying this healthy and delicious meal.

You can always customize this recipe by adding your favorite herbs and spices, or other vegetables of your choice. The simplicity of this dish makes it perfect for a quick weeknight dinner or entertaining guests. With delicious flavor and health benefits, baked salmon with dill and asparagus is sure to become a favorite on your meal plan.

Quinoa stuffed peppers

Quinoa stuffed peppers combine a blend of colorful peppers, protein-rich quinoa, and flavorful ingredients to create a nutritious and filling dish. Featured in the Sprint Count Calories Cookbook for Fledglings, this recipe offers a delicious and healthy option for any vegetarian or vegan diet.

To prepare quinoa stuffed peppers:

Material
4 bell peppers (any color), stems, and seeds removed.
1 cup quinoa (washed)

2 cups vegetable broth or water

1 tablespoon olive oil

1 small onion (chopped)

2 garlic cloves (chopped)

1 zucchini, diced

1 carrot, diced

1/2 cup corn kernels (fresh or frozen)

1/2 cup black beans (washed and drained)

1/2 cup diced tomatoes

1 teaspoon dried oregano

1 teaspoon powdered cumin

salt and pepper to taste

Discretionary fixings

Destroyed cheese, chopped new cilantro, cut avocado, salsa.

Enlightening

Warm the olive oil in a gigantic skillet or wok over medium-high heat.

Incorporate the shrimp in the skillet and cook for 2-3 minutes per side, until they turn pink and dull. Be careful not to overcook the shrimp, as they can get rubbery. Oust the cooked shrimp from the skillet and set aside.

Combine quinoa and vegetable stock or water in a medium-sized pan. Bring to a bubble over medium warm. Decrease warm, cover, and stew until quinoa is delicate and fluid is retained, approximately 15-20 minutes. Remove from the stove and let it stand for some minutes with the cover on. Remove from the heat and let it sit secured for many minutes.

Within the between times, warm the olive oil in a colossal skillet over medium warm. Include the diced onion and minced garlic, and sauté for 2-3 minutes until they become fragrant and translucent.

Include the diced zucchini, carrot, corn parts, dark beans, diced tomatoes, dried oregano, and ground cumin in the skillet. Season with salt and pepper to taste. Broil for another 5-7 minutes until the vegetables are delicate.

Once the quinoa is cooked and marginally cooled, include it in the skillet with the sautéed vegetables. Blend well to combine all the fixings. Alter the flavoring in case required.

Spoon the quinoa and vegetable blend into the emptied chime peppers, squeezing tenderly to fill them equally. Put the tops back on the chime peppers, making a seal.

Heat the stuffed chime peppers on the preheated stove for around 25-30 minutes, or until the peppers are delicate and marginally charred. Cooking time may change depending on the size and thickness of the peppers.

After cooking is total, expel the stuffed peppers from the oven and permit them to cool somewhat sometime recently.

Serve the quinoa stuffed chime peppers hot, alternatively topped with destroyed cheese, chopped new cilantro, cut avocado, or salsa.

These fixings incorporate extra flavor and surface to the dish.

Quinoa-stuffed chime peppers make for a well-balanced and fulfilling supper that's stuffed with fiber, vitamins, and minerals. The "Sprint Number Calories Cookbook for Juveniles" may give serving recommendations and dietary data to help fledglings in following their caloric admissions successfully whereas getting a charge out of this delightful and nutritious dish.

Feel free to test with distinctive vegetables, herbs, or flavors to suit your taste preferences. These stuffed chime peppers can be delighted in as a standalone supper or combined with a new serving of mixed greens or whole-grain bread for a total and fulfilling feasting involvement.

Chapter 4

Week by week Supper Arrange with Moo Sodium Formulas

Week 1:

Flavorful Moo Sodium Suppers

Within the "Sprint Tally Calories Cookbook for Juveniles," Week 1 is committed to presenting flavorful moo sodium suppers that are both tasty and careful of your well-being. This week's feast arranges centers on lessening sodium admissions whereas still joining an assortment of flavors and fixings to keep your taste buds fulfilled.

Here's a test dinner arrange for Week 1:

Day 1:
Herb-Roasted Chicken with Steamed Vegetables
Begin the week with a flavorful herb-roasted chicken dish. Season the chicken with a mix of herbs, such as rosemary, thyme, and garlic powder, and cook it until it's succulent and delicate. Serve with steamed vegetables such as broccoli, carrots, and cauliflower. This feast is moo in sodium, tall in protein, and stuffed with basic supplements.

Day 2:
Quinoa Stuffed Chime Peppers
Appreciate a vegan feast with quinoa stuffed chime peppers. The chime peppers are filled with a blend of quinoa, sautéed vegetables, and flavorful herbs and flavors. Cook them until the peppers are delicate and the filling is hot. This

dish isn't as it were low in sodium but moreover wealthy in fiber and vitamins.

Day 3:
Lemon Garlic Shrimp Stir-Fry
Enjoy a lively and moo sodium stir-fry with lemon garlic shrimp. Sauté the shrimp with garlic, lemon pizzazz, and new lemon juice for a burst of citrusy flavor. Include a colorful blend of stir-fried vegetables like chime peppers, snap peas, and carrots. Serve it over brown rice or quinoa for a well-balanced dinner.

Day 4:
Heated Salmon with Dill and Asparagus
Savor a heart-healthy dish of prepared salmon with dill and asparagus. Season the salmon with new dill, lemon juice, and a touch of olive oil, at that point heat it until it's flaky and wet. Match it with simmered asparagus for a nutritious and moo sodium supper alternative.

Day 5:
Barbecued Angle Tacos with New Salsa

Flavor up your Friday night with flame-broiled angle tacos with new salsa. Flame broil white angle filets with a flavorful zest rub, at that point, serve them in warm corn tortillas. Beat the angle with a hand-crafted salsa made from diced tomatoes, ruddy onions, cilantro, and a press of lime juice. These angle tacos are moo in sodium and pressed with dynamic flavors.

Day 6:

Quinoa Serving of mixed greens with Roasted Vegetables and Feta Cheese

Appreciate reviving a quinoa serving of mixed greens stuffed with simmered vegetables and disintegrated feta cheese. Broil an assortment of vegetables, such as chime peppers, zucchini, and eggplant, at that point, hurl them with cooked quinoa and disintegrated feta cheese. Sprinkle with a light vinaigrette for additional flavor

Day 7:

Lentil Soup with Whole Wheat Bread
End the week with a comforting homemade lentil soup. Boil lentils in a low-salt vegetable broth with flavorful vegetables like onions, carrots, and celery. Seasoning with herbs such as thyme or bay leaf will add more flavor. Eating soup with whole-grain bread will fill you up.

By incorporating these delicious low-sodium meals into your week 1 meal plan, you can experiment with different flavors while keeping your salt intake under control.

The Sprint Count Calories Cookbook for Chicks includes detailed recipes and nutritional information for each dish to help beginners strive for healthier eating habits. Adjust servings to meet specific dietary needs and consult a healthcare professional if you have specific health concerns. Enjoy delicious, low-sodium meals all week long.

Second week:
Quick and easy-low salt dinner

Week 2 of the Sprint Count Calories Cookbook for Chicks focuses on showing you convenient, delicious, quick, and easy low-sodium dinner options. These meals are designed to save you time in the kitchen while providing delicious, nutritious meals.

Here's a case feast arrange for Week 2:

First day:
Pan-fried Lemon and Herb Chicken with Vegetables
Start the week with an easy and hearty one-pan dish. Mix chicken breast with lemon zest, herbs such as thyme and rosemary, and season with a little olive oil. Place the chicken on a baking sheet along with colorful vegetables such as potatoes, carrots, and Brussels sprouts. Roast

everything in the oven until the chicken is cooked through and the vegetables are tender and caramelized.

The 2nd day:
Turkey and Vegetable Skillet
Enjoy a quick and delicious turkey and veggie bun. Sauté ground turkey with garlic, ginger, and low-salt pan sauce. Add colorful vegetables such as peppers, broccoli, and mangoes. Serve the skillet with brown rice or whole-grain pasta for a balanced and hearty dinner.

Third day:
Spaghetti squash with tomato basil sauce
Replace regular pasta with spaghetti squash for a low-sodium alternative. Bake the spaghetti squash in the oven until tender and scrape out the fibers. Served with homemade tomato basil sauce made with diced tomatoes, fresh basil, garlic, and olive oil. A sprinkle of grated Parmesan cheese adds more flavor.

Day 4:

Grilled cod with herb quinoa pilaf
Make a light, fluffy grilled cod fillet and pair it with flavorful quinoa pilaf. Season the cod with herbs, lemon juice, and a little olive oil, and bake in the oven until slightly crumbled. Quinoa is cooked and tossed with a blend of herbs and spices such as sautéed onions, garlic, parsley, thyme, and paprika. Serve cod over herb-infused quinoa pilaf for a nutritious and filling meal.

Day 5:
Teriyaki Vegetable and Tofu Stir-Fry
Appreciate a vegan stir-fried with a scrumptious teriyaki turn. Sauté tofu 3d shapes with a variety of colorful vegetables such as chime peppers, broccoli, and carrots. Sprinkle the stir-fried with a custom-made moo sodium teriyaki sauce made from soy sauce, nectar, ginger, and garlic. Serve it with brown rice or quinoa for a total and flavorful supper.

Day 6:

Lemon Herb Flame broiled Chicken Sticks with a Mediterranean Serving of mixed greens

Fire up the flame-broil and get ready lemon herb flame broiled chicken sticks. Marinate chicken pieces in a blend of lemon juice, herbs like oregano and thyme, and olive oil. Stick chicken and flame-broil until delicately browned. Serve the chicken sticks nearby a reviving Mediterranean serving of mixed greens made with cucumbers, tomatoes, ruddy onions, olives, and feta cheese.

Day 7:

Vegetable and Bean Soup with Entirety Grain Bread

Conclude the week with a comforting and feeding vegetable and bean soup. Stew an assortment of vegetables such as carrots, celery, onions, and diced tomatoes in a moo sodium vegetable broth. Include your favorite beans like cannellini or dark beans for protein and fiber. Season the soup with herbs and flavors like inlet clears out, thyme, and dark pepper. Serve it with a cut of entire-grain bread for a fulfilling supper. By joining these fast and simple moo sodium meals in your Week 2 feast arrangement, you'll be able to appreciate tasty and nutritious suppers without investing

Week 3:
Family-Friendly Low Sodium Formulas
Within the "Sprint Check Calories Cookbook for Juveniles," Week 3 centers on family-friendly moo sodium formulas that are beyond any doubt if you don't mind both kids and grown-ups alike. These recipes are planned to be flavorful, nutritious, and agreeable for the total family.

Here's a test feast arrange for Week 3:

Day 1:
Oven-Baked Chicken Chunks with Sweet Potato Fries
Kick off the week with a more advantageous bend on a family favorite. Plan oven-baked chicken pieces utilizing inclined chicken breast,

entire wheat breadcrumbs, and an assortment of herbs and flavors. Serve them with hand-crafted sweet potato fries, prepared with a touch of olive oil and your favorite herbs.

Day 2:
Vegetable Lasagna with Entirety Wheat Noodles
Assemble the family around for comforting and moo sodium vegetable lasagna. Layer entire wheat lasagna noodles with a blend of sautéed vegetables like zucchini, chime peppers, spinach, and mushrooms. Utilize moo-sodium marinara sauce and moo fat ricotta cheese to keep it nutritious and flavorful.

Day 3:
Turkey Meatballs with Marinara Sauce and Spaghetti
Appreciate a classic favorite with a more advantageous bend. Make turkey meatballs utilizing inclined ground turkey, entirely wheat breadcrumbs, and an assortment of herbs and flavors. Serve the meatballs over the entirety of

the wheat spaghetti with a custom-made marinara sauce made from moo sodium canned tomatoes, garlic, and herbs.

Day 4:

Dark Bean and Vegetable Quesadillas

Get imaginative with a family-friendly feast of dark bean and vegetable quesadillas. Squash dark beans and blend them with sautéed vegetables like chime peppers, onions, and corn. Spread the blend onto entire wheat tortillas, sprinkle with reduced-fat cheese, and cook until brilliant and firm.

Day 5:

Teriyaki Salmon with Stir-Fried Vegetables and Brown Rice

Present your family with the flavors of teriyaki with this nutritious supper. Marinate salmon fillets in a moo sodium teriyaki sauce, at that point flame broil or prepare them until they're flaky and delightful. Serve the salmon with a side of stir-fried vegetables, such as broccoli, snap peas, carrots, and chime peppers, and steamed brown rice for a total and fulfilling supper.

Day 6:
Turkey Taco Lettuce Wraps
Make taco night a more advantageous issue with turkey taco lettuce wraps. Cook ground turkey with taco flavoring and serve it wrapped in fresh lettuce. Offer an assortment of garnishes like diced tomatoes, avocado, moo fat cheese, and Greek yogurt for a customizable and family-friendly supper.

Day 7:
Veggie Pizza with Entire Wheat Hull
Concluding the week with a fun and intelligent supper of veggie pizza. Utilize a whole wheat pizza outside as the base and let everybody within the family select their favorite moo sodium fixings, such as sautéed vegetables, cut tomatoes, olives, and reduced-fat cheese. Heat until the mixture is firm and the cheese is dissolved.

By joining these family-friendly moo sodium formulas into your Week 3 dinner arrangement, you'll guarantee that your whole family can appreciate scrumptious and nutritious suppers together. The "Sprint Tally Calories Cookbook for Juveniles" may give nitty gritty formulas and serving proposals to help tenderfoots in following their caloric admissions while savoring these delicious dishes. Feel free to customize the formulas to suit your family's inclinations, and appreciate the holding time that comes with planning and sharing dinners together.

Week 4:

Veggie lover and Vegetarian Moo Sodium Alternatives

Within the "Sprint Tally Calories Cookbook for Juveniles," Week 4 is committed to vegan and vegetarian moo sodium alternatives. These formulas are pressed with plant-based goodness, giving an assortment of flavors, surfaces, and supplements. Whether you take after a vegan or vegetarian way of life or essentially need to join more meatless suppers into your count calories, this week's feast offers scrumptious and fulfilling choices.

Here's a test dinner arrange for Week 4:

Day 1:
Chickpea and Vegetable Curry
Begin the week with a flavorful and nutritious chickpea and vegetable curry. Sauté a blend of vegetables such as chime peppers, carrots, and cauliflower with fragrant flavors like curry powder, turmeric, and cumin. Add cooked chickpeas and coconut drain for creaminess. Serve the curry over brown rice or quinoa for a total and fulfilling feast.

Day 2:
Lentil and Vegetable Stir-Fry
Appreciate a protein-packed lentil and vegetable stir-fry. Sauté an assortment of colorful vegetables like broccoli, snow peas, and chime peppers with cooked lentils and a moo sodium stir-fry sauce. Serve it over brown rice or

entirely wheat noodles for a well-rounded and flavorful supper.

Day 3:
Caprese Serving of mixed greens with Balsamic Coat
Enchant in a reviving and moo sodium Caprese serving of mixed greens. Layer cuts of ready tomatoes and new mozzarella cheese, at that point, decorate with new basil, and clear out. Sprinkle with a tart balsamic coat for included flavor. This basic, however rich serving of mixed greens is idealized as a light lunch or a side dish.

Day 4:
Spinach and Mushroom Stuffed Portobello Mushrooms
Get inventive with stuffed portobello mushrooms filled with a flavorful spinach and mushroom blend. Sauté spinach, mushrooms, onions, and garlic, at that point, blend in breadcrumbs and ground Parmesan cheese. Stuff the blend into portobello mushroom caps and

prepare until the mushrooms are delicate and the filling is brilliant brown.

Day 5:

Vegetarian Lentil Tacos with Avocado Crema

Appreciate a meatless bend on taco night with veggie lover lentil tacos. Cook lentils with flavors like cumin, paprika, and chili powder, at that point utilize them as a filling for taco shells or lettuce wraps. Beat together with your favorite taco fixings such as diced tomatoes, avocado cuts, and a hand-crafted avocado crema made from mixed avocado, lime juice, and a touch of salt.

Day 6:

Quinoa and Dark Bean Serving of mixed greens with Lime Dressing

Plan a reviving and protein-rich quinoa and dark bean serving of mixed greens. Cook quinoa and blend it with dark beans, colorful vegetables like chime peppers and corn, and a fiery lime dressing made from new lime juice, olive oil, and herbs. This serving of mixed greens can be delighted in as a primary dish or served as a side of nearby barbecued vegetables or tofu.

Day 7:
Sweet Potato and Chickpea Buddha Bowl
Conclude the week with feeding and fulfilling sweet potato and chickpea Buddha bowl. Broil sweet potato 3d shapes and chickpeas with a sprinkle of cumin and paprika until they're firm and brilliant. Serve them over a bed of cooked quinoa or brown rice, and include an assortment of new vegetables like cucumber, avocado, and cherry tomatoes. Sprinkle with a tahini dressing for additional creaminess.

By consolidating these vegan and vegetarian moo sodium choices into your Week 4 super arrangement, you can enjoy a different run of plant-based suppers that are both nutritious and delightful. The "Sprint Number Calories Cookbook for Juveniles" may give point-by-point formulas and wholesome data for each dish to help tenderfoots in following their caloric admissions while investigating these flavorful meatless choices. Feel free to alter the formula to suit your taste inclinations and dietary needs. Try distinctive herbs, flavors, and vegetables to include an assortment and find modern flavors. These veggie lover and veggie lover moo sodium choices are not as useful for your well-being but moreover contribute to a more maintainable and ecologically inviting way of life. Appreciate the wealth of plant-based fixings and the feeding suppers they make.

Week 5:

Delightful Moo Sodium Consolation Nourishments

Within the "Sprint Tally Calories Cookbook for Juveniles," Week 5 is all approximately fulfilling your longings for comforting and delightful suppers whereas keeping sodium levels in check. These formulas offer a more advantageous bend on classic consolation nourishments, giving warmth, flavor, and fulfillment without compromising your dietary objectives. Get prepared to enjoy guilt-free consultation with this test feast arranged for Week 5:

Day 1:
Butternut Squash Soup
Start the week with a bowl of velvety and flavorful butternut squash soup. Broil butternut squash with onions and garlic until delicate, at that point mix it with moo sodium vegetable broth until smooth. Season with herbs and flavors like nutmeg and thyme for a comforting and feeding soup.

Day 2:
Turkey Chili
Appreciate a generous and moo sodium turkey chili pressed with protein and flavor. Brown incline ground turkey with onions, garlic, and a mix of chili flavors. Include kidney beans, diced tomatoes, and moo sodium tomato sauce, at that point stew until the flavors merge together.

Serve with a spot of Greek yogurt and a sprinkle of new herbs for included freshness.

Day 3:
Prepared Mac and Cheese with Cauliflower
Treat yourself to a healthier version of the classic mac and cheese by adding cauliflower for extra nutrition and creaminess. Whole-wheat macaroni is cooked al dente and tossed with a cheese sauce made from low-sodium cheese, Greek yogurt, and a dash of Dijon mustard. Stir in the steamed cauliflower florets and bake until golden and bubbly.

Day 4:
Peppers stuffed with lean ground meat
Enjoy stuffed peppers with a flavorful blend of lean ground meat, quinoa, onions, and a variety of vegetables. Flavor the filling with herbs and spices such as oregano and paprika. Bake the pepper stuffing until the peppers are soft and the

insides are cooked through. Serve with a side salad for a hearty meal.

Day 5:
Vegetable pot pie
Enjoy a convenient veggie pot pie with no added salt. Sauté a mixture of vegetables such as carrots, peas, corn, and potatoes in low-sodium vegetable broth until tender. Make a creamy sauce by mixing the low-salt milk and flour and pouring it over the vegetables. Top with a sheet of whole wheat dough or a layer of mashed cauliflower and bake until golden brown and bubbly.

Day 6:
Oven-baked chicken parmesan cheese
Satisfy your Italian food cravings with our healthier Chicken Parmesan. Chicken breast is coated with wholemeal breadcrumbs seasoned with herbs and spices and baked in the oven until golden brown and cooked through. Drizzle

with low-salt marinara sauce and sprinkle with low-salt mozzarella cheese. Serve with whole-grain spaghetti or zucchini noodles for a pleasantly balanced dinner.

Day 7:
Banana Bread Oatmeal
End the week on a sweet note with a cup of warm and comforting Banana Bread Oatmeal. Add mashed bananas, cinnamon, and maple syrup to the oats and simmer until creamy and fragrant. Sprinkle with chopped walnuts or almonds for extra crunchiness and a little almond butter for extra texture.

By incorporating these delicious, low-sodium, feel-good foods into your Week 5 meal plan, you can enjoy the joys of classic cooking while keeping your health goals in mind.

The Sprint Count Calories Cookbook for Beginners includes detailed recipes and serving suggestions to help beginners keep track of their calorie intake while enjoying these beneficial meals. Feel free to adjust the recipe to suit your taste preferences and dietary needs, and enjoy the nutritious and filling taste of these comfort foods without compromising your health.

Chapter 5

31-Day Dinner Arrangement for Bringing Down Blood Weight

Keeping up sound blood weight is exceptionally critical for by and large well-being and lessening the chance of cardiovascular illness. One critical figure that impacts blood weight levels is counting calories. The nourishments we devour can either contribute to tall blood weight (hypertension) or offer assistance to oversee and lower it. In this area of the "Sprint Check Calories Cookbook for Juveniles," we'll investigate the association between blood weight and diet, providing you with profitable data to create educated choices around your eating propensities.

Understanding Blood Weight

Blood weight is the constraint the heart applies on the dividers of supply routes because it pumps blood through the body. It is measured in millimeters of mercury (mmHg) and consists of two values:

Systolic and diastolic blood weight.

systolic weight and diastolic weight.

The systolic weight speaks to the constraints when the heart contracts, whereas the diastolic weight is the drive when the heart is at rest between beats. A blood weight of around 120/80 mmHg is for the most part considered ordinary.

The Effect of Slim Down on Blood Weight:

A slim-down tall in sodium (salt) could be a well-known supporter of tall blood weight. Over-the-top sodium admissions can lead to liquid maintenance, expanded blood volume, and hoisted blood weight. In any case, it's not fair sodium that influences blood pressure—other supplements and dietary designs play a part as well.

Here are a few imperative dietary variables to consider:

Sodium

Constraining sodium admissions is key to overseeing blood weight. The suggested daily sodium admissions for grown-ups is ordinarily around 2,300 milligrams (mg) or less. Diminishing handled and bundled nourishments, which tend to be tall in sodium, and opting for new, whole foods could be a great procedure.

Potassium

Devouring nourishments wealthy in potassium can offer assistance offset the impacts of sodium and lower blood weight. Great sources of potassium incorporate natural products, bananas, oranges, avocados, vegetables, spinach, sweet potatoes, tomatoes, vegetables beans, and lentils.

Magnesium

Satisfactory magnesium admissions are related to lower blood weight. Nourishments such as verdant greens, nuts and seeds, entirety grains, and vegetables are amazing sources of magnesium.

Fiber

A high-fiber eat less, especially one wealthy in dissolvable fiber, has been shown to assist in diminishing blood weight. Incorporate entire grains, natural products, vegetables, and legumes in your suppers to extend your fiber admissions.

Sound Fats

Pick unsaturated fats found in nourishments like avocados, olive oil, nuts, and seeds. These fats have been related to a diminished hazard of tall blood weight and cardiovascular infections.

Adjusted Count calories
Taking after a well-balanced eat-less that incorporates an assortment of natural products, vegetables, entirety grains, incline proteins, and sound fats can contribute to general heart well-being and offer assistance to oversee blood pressure levels.

Within the "Sprint Number Calories Cookbook for Juveniles," will offer you a range of delightful, moo sodium formulas that join nutrient-rich fixings to bolster a sound blood weight. By understanding the effect of eating less on blood weight and making cognizant choices around the nourishments you expend, you'll take critical steps toward advancing heart well-being and keeping up ideal blood weight levels. Continuously counsel along with your healthcare supplier or an enrolled dietitian for personalized counsel and direction with respect to your particular dietary needs and well-being conditions.

Day 1
Heart-Healthy Formulas for Breakfast, Lunch, and Supper

To kick off your week on a heart-healthy note, we have curated a choice of nutritious and delightful formulas for breakfast, lunch, and supper. These formulas are moo in sodium, wealthy in basic supplements, and planned to back your cardiovascular well-being. Let's jump into the heavenly alternatives for each dinner of the day.

Breakfast

Begin your day with a heart-healthy breakfast that powers your body and fulfills your taste buds.

Choice 1
Veggie Omelet

Whisk together egg whites and a splash of low-fat drain. Cook the blend in a non-stick skillet and fill it with a grouping of colorful vegetables like spinach, chime peppers, and tomatoes. Best with a sprinkle of low-sodium feta cheese for included flavor.

Alternative 2
Overnight Chia Pudding
Combine chia seeds with a low-fat drains or plant-based drain, such as an almond or soy drain, in a jar. Add a touch of nectar or maple syrup for sweetness and mix well. Refrigerate overnight and best with new berries and a sprinkle of chopped nuts in the morning.

Lunch
Keep your late-morning supper light, flavorful, and heart-healthy with these fulfilling alternatives.

Choice 1

Grilled Chicken and Quinoa Serving of mixed greens

Flame broil, incline chicken breast, and cut it into strips. Hurl cooked quinoa with an assortment of new vegetables like cucumbers, cherry tomatoes, and blended greens. Sprinkle with a custom-made vinaigrette made with olive oil, lemon juice, and herbs.

Alternative 2

Mediterranean Chickpea Serving of mixed greens
Combine cooked chickpeas with diced cucumber, cherry tomatoes, ruddy onion, and Kalamata olives. Dress the serving of mixed greens with a blend of lemon juice, olive oil, garlic, and dried herbs like oregano and basil. Best with disintegrated low-sodium feta cheese for an additional tart kick.

Supper

Wrap up your day with a heart-healthy supper that's both nourishing and fulfilling.

Alternative 1

Heated Salmon with Lemon-Dill Sauce

Place a fresh salmon filet on a preparing sheet and season it with herbs, such as dill and thyme, in conjunction with a crush of lemon juice. Prepare until the salmon is cooked and cushy. Serve with a side of broiled asparagus and a velvety lemon-dill sauce.

Alternative 2

Lentil and Vegetable Stir-Fry

Sauté a variety of colorful vegetables like chime peppers, broccoli, and snap peas in a non-stick skillet. Include cooked lentils and a low-sodium stir-fry sauce made from soy sauce, ginger, and garlic. In the event that you put brown rice or quinoa on a searing skillet and eat it, you'll appreciate a generous supper.

These heart-healthy formulas for breakfast, lunch, and supper give an adjusted and flavorful approach to advancing cardiovascular well-being. They are a test of the numerous nutritious alternatives accessible within the "Sprint Check Calories Cookbook for Juveniles." Explore diverse fixings, herbs, and flavors to customize the recipes to your taste inclinations and dietary needs. Keep in mind to enroll a dietitian for personalized direction on overseeing your heart wellbeing and dietary prerequisites. Appreciate these feeding dinners and embrace a heart-healthy way of life!

Day 7-13

Low-Sodium Snacks and Refreshments

Within the "Sprint Calories Cookbook for Juveniles," we get the significance of keeping up a low-sodium count of calories all through the day, counting nibble time. Snacks and refreshments can frequently contribute a critical sum of sodium to our every day admissions, so it's fundamental to create careful choices. Here are a few flavorful and low-sodium alternatives for snacks and refreshments to appreciate amid days 7 to 13:

Snacks

Snacking can be both pleasant and nutritious with these low-sodium choices:

Day 7
New Natural product Serving of mixed greens
Create a reviving natural product serving of mixed greens employing an assortment of regular natural products like berries, melons, and citrus. Hurl the natural products together and include a crush of lime or lemon juice for an additional burst of flavor. This actually sweet and colorful nibble is stuffed with vitamins and cancer-prevention agents.

Day 8
Homemade Hummus and Veggies

Whip up a clump of custom-made hummus utilizing low-sodium canned chickpeas, garlic, lemon juice, and tahini. Combine it with a grouping of colorful cut vegetables like carrots, cucumbers, and chime peppers. This combination gives fiber, protein, and basic supplements whereas fulfilling your nibble longings.

Day 9
Greek Yogurt with Berries and Almonds
Appreciate a serving of low-sodium Greek yogurt topped with a modest bunch of new berries and a sprinkle of chopped almonds. This snack offers a rich surface, an implication of sweetness, and a fulfilling crunch. Greek yogurt is wealthy in protein, whereas berries and almonds give cancer prevention agents and sound fats.

Day 10
Rice Cakes with Avocado and Tomato

Spread a lean layer of mashed avocado on a low-sodium rice cake and beat it with cut tomatoes. Sprinkle a squeeze of ocean salt or a sodium-free flavoring mix for included flavor. This nibble is light, crunchy, and pressed with solid monounsaturated fats from the avocado.
Refreshments:

Remain hydrated and taste these moo sodium refreshments all through the week:

Day 11
Implanted Water with Cucumber and Mint
Improve your hydration with a reviving cucumber and mint-infused water. Include cut cucumbers and a number of sprigs of new mint in a pitcher of water and let it imbue within the fridge. This calorie-free and reviving refreshment could be an idealized way to extinguish your thirst.

Day 12
Herbal iced tea

Prepare a pot of herbal tea with your favorite flavors, such as chamomile, peppermint, or hibiscus. Refrigerate until cold. A squeeze of lemon or a sprig of fresh mint in iced tea makes for a delicious and comforting drink.

Day 13
freshly squeezed citrus juice
Squeeze the juice of fresh orange, grapefruit, or lemon for a vibrant, invigorating citrus drink. Dilute with water if desired and add a bit of a natural sweetener such as honey or stevia. Citrus juices are rich in vitamin C and provide a refreshing taste.

These low-sodium snacks and drinks offer a delicious way to satisfy your appetite while controlling your sodium intake. Feel free to adjust the recipe to your taste and experiment with different fruits, vegetables, and herbs. Enjoy these snacks and drinks as part of a balanced and nutritious diet. Remember, it's important to seek individual advice from your doctor or registered dietitian about managing your sodium intake and overall health. Cheers to your health and happiness!

Days 14-20
Hearty salads and soups
Continuing the Sprint Count Calories Cookbook for Fledgling's nutritious eating journey, we present a selection of salads and soups that will nourish your body and satisfy your taste buds from day 14 to day 20. These recipes are designed to manage your sodium intake while providing a variety of essential nutrients such as vitamins, minerals, fiber, and antioxidants. Explore delicious salad and soup options this time of year.

Day 14
Caprese salad
Arrange ripe tomato slices, fresh mozzarella cheese, and basil leaves on a plate. Sprinkle with additional virgin olive oil and balsamic coat. Sprinkle some salt and black pepper over it. This classic Italian salad is flavorful and rich in vitamins and calcium.

Day 15

Asian coleslaw

Julienne kale, red cabbage, julienne carrots, and slice leeks. Toss the vegetables with a dressing that includes low-salt soy sauce, rice vinegar, sesame oil, and a little honey. Decorate with toasted sesame seeds for included surface and flavor.

Day 16

Beet and goat cheese salad

Roast or steam the beets until tender and slice thinly. Arrange the beets on a bed of mixed vegetables, sprinkle with goat cheese, and sprinkle with chopped walnuts. Drizzle with a light dressing of olive oil, lemon juice, and Dijon mustard soup:

Day 17

Tomato Basil Soup

Sauté diced onions and minced garlic in olive oil until relaxed. Include canned diced tomatoes, vegetable broth, and a modest bunch of new basil clear-out. Stew until the flavors merge together, at that point mix the blend until smooth. Include a squeeze of salt and dark pepper to taste. Sprinkle with ground parmesan and serve.

Day 18
Moroccan Lentil Soup

In a pot, combine cooked lentils, diced tomatoes, chopped carrots, celery, onions, and a mix of Moroccan flavors like cumin, coriander, and cinnamon. Stew until the vegetables are delicate and the flavors are implanted. This healthy soup is wealthy in protein, fiber, and warm flavors.

Day 19
Rich Broccoli Soup

Steam or bubble new broccoli until delicate. Mix the broccoli with vegetable broth, low-fat drain or non-dairy drain, and impurity of garlic powder. Include a squeeze of salt and dark pepper to taste. For included creaminess, mix in a spot of Greek yogurt or a sprinkle of wholesome yeast.

Day 20
Chicken and Vegetable Noodle Soup
Stew chicken breast, cut carrots, celery, onions, and low-sodium chicken broth in a pot until the chicken is cooked through and the vegetables are delicate. Shred the chicken and return it to the pot alongside the cooked noodles. Season with herbs like thyme and parsley for additional flavor.

These nutrient-packed servings of mixed greens and soups give a feeding and delightful way to consolidate an assortment of vitamins, minerals, and fiber into your day-by-day dinners. Customize the formulas by including your favorite vegetables, herbs, or flavors to suit your taste inclinations. Keep in mind to select low-sodium fixings and restrain included salt for heart-healthy alternatives. Appreciate these flavorful and fulfilling servings of mixed greens and soups as a portion of your adjusted and nutrient-rich eating arrangement.

Day 21-27
Incline Protein and Entire Grain Suppers

Within the "Sprint Calories Cookbook for Juveniles," we proceed our travel towards more beneficial eating with a center on lean protein and entire grains from days 21 to 27. These dinners are planned to supply fundamental supplements, advance satiety, and bolster yours by and large well-being. Let's investigate a few flavorful and fulfilling formulas that join incline protein and entirety grains into your count calories.

Day 21
Barbecued Chicken Breast with Quinoa and Roasted Vegetables

Barbecue is a skinless chicken breast prepared with herbs and flavors of your choice. Serve it nearby a parcel of cooked quinoa and a medley of simmered vegetables such as broccoli, chime peppers, and zucchini. This supper is pressed with incline protein, fiber-rich quinoa, and a cluster of vitamins and minerals from the vegetables.

Day 22
Prepared Salmon with Brown Rice and Steamed Asparagus

Heat a new salmon filet prepared with lemon juice, garlic, and herbs. Combine it with a serving of cooked brown rice and softly steamed asparagus lances. This dish gives heart-healthy omega-3 greasy acids from the salmon, fiber from the brown rice, and basic supplements from the asparagus.

Day 23
Turkey Lettuce Wraps with Quinoa Serving of mixed greens

Get ready for flavorful turkey lettuce wraps by sautéing incline ground turkey with onions, garlic, and Asian-inspired seasonings. Wrap the turkey blend in huge lettuce clears out and serve with a reviving quinoa serving of mixed greens blended with diced cucumbers, cherry tomatoes, and a light vinaigrette dressing. This dinner offers inclined protein, entire grains, and dosage of new vegetables.

Day 24
Dark Bean and Vegetable Stir-Fry with Brown Rice
Sauté a blend of colorful vegetables like chime peppers, broccoli, carrots, and snap peas with dark beans in a light stir-fry sauce. Serve the stir-fry over a bed of cooked brown rice for a total and fulfilling feast. This dish is rich in plant-based protein, fiber, and an assortment of vitamins and minerals.

Day 25
Flame-broiled Shrimp Sticks with Quinoa and Barbecued Vegetables
Stick expansive shrimp marinated in a fiery mix of lemon juice, garlic, and flavors, at that point flame broil until cooked through. Serve the shrimp sticks with a side of cooked quinoa and an assortment of flame-broiled vegetables such as eggplant, zucchini, and chime peppers. This

feast gives inclined protein from shrimp, entire grains from quinoa, and a mixture of flame-broiled vegetables for included flavor and supplements.

Day 26

Heated Chicken Thighs with Wild Rice Pilaf and Simmered Brussels Grows

Prepare skinless chicken thighs prepared with herbs and flavors until brilliant and fresh. Serve the chicken thighs with a side of wild rice pilaf and roasted Brussels sprouts. This dish offers incline protein from the chicken, fiber-rich wild rice, and liberal measurements of vitamins and minerals from the Brussels sprouts.

Day 27

Lentil and Vegetable Curry with Quinoa

Cook a flavorful lentil and vegetable curry employing an assortment of vegetables, lentils, and fragrant flavors. Serve the curry over a bed of cooked quinoa for a total and feeding dinner. This dish is stuffed with plant-based protein, fiber, and a cluster of vitamins and minerals.

These incline protein and entirety grain dinners give an adjusted combination of supplements, advancing satiety, and supporting your by and large wellbeing and well-being. Feel free to customize the formulas by including your favorite herbs, flavors, or vegetables to suit your taste inclinations. Keep in mind to select incline cuts of protein, pick entire grain assortments, and hone parcel control for a well-rounded and nutritious eating arrangement.

Day 28-34

Plant-Based Alternatives for a Healthy Heart

Within the "Sprint Tally Calories Cookbook for Juveniles," we set out on a journey towards heart-healthy eating with a center on plant-based alternatives from days 28 to 34. Joining plant-based dinners into your count calories can give various well-being benefits, counting progressed heart well-being, expanded fiber admissions, and decreased chance of incessant maladies. Let's investigate a few flavorful and nutritious plant-based formulas that will feed your body and back a solid heart.

Day 28

Chickpea and Vegetable Curry

Get ready for a scrumptious curry by stewing chickpeas, blended vegetables such as chime peppers, cauliflower, and peas, and fragrant flavors in a tomato-based sauce. Serve the curry over a bed of brown rice or quinoa for a total and fulfilling dinner. This dish is wealthy in plant-based protein, fiber, and a cluster of vitamins and minerals.

Day 29

Lentil walnut burger and sweet potato fries

Combine cooked lentils, finely chopped walnuts, whole grain bread crumbs, and flavorful seasonings to create a homemade veggie burger. Form patties from the mixture and bake or grill until firm and golden brown. A lentil and walnut burger is placed in a whole wheat bun and garnished with freshly baked sweet potato fries.

This diet includes plant-based protein, heart-healthy fats, and a variety of essential nutrients.

Day 30

Quinoa salad with roasted vegetables

A mixture of roasted vegetables such as eggplant, zucchini, bell peppers, and cherry tomatoes is mixed with cooked quinoa and a tangy vinaigrette dressing. Add fresh herbs such as parsley or basil for added flavor. This salad is rich in fiber, vitamins, minerals, and antioxidants.

Day 31

Black bean tacos with avocado salsa

Soft corn tortillas are stuffed with a bright avocado salsa made with seasoned black beans, sautéed peppers, onions, diced avocado, tomatoes, red onions, cilantro, lime juice, and a pinch of salt. These delicious, filling tacos are packed with plant-based protein, fiber, and healthy fats.

Day 32

Vegan lentil and vegetable bread

Colorful vegetables such as broccoli, carrots, snow peas, and green peppers are lightly stir-fried with low-salt soy sauce, garlic, and ginger. Add cooked lentils as a vegetable protein and stir-fry and serve over brown rice or quinoa.

Day 33

Portobello mushroom stuffed with spinach and mushrooms

Stuff a large portobello mushroom umbrella with a mixture of sautéed spinach, mushrooms, onions, garlic, and bread crumbs. Prepare until the mushrooms are delicate and the filling is brilliant brown. These flavorful mushroom fillings are packed with vitamins, minerals, and fiber.

Day 34

Buddha bowl with quinoa and roasted vegetables

Combine cooked quinoa, roasted vegetables such as sweet potatoes, Brussels sprouts, cauliflower, leafy greens, and a dash of tahini dressing for a nutritious Buddha bowl. This healthy bowl contains a variety of nutrients including fiber, protein, and healthy fats.

These plant-based, heart-healthy options offer a variety of flavors, textures, and essential nutrients that support good health. Eating a plant-based diet not only contributes to cardiovascular health but also promotes sustainability and reduces your carbon footprint. You can always customize your recipe by adding your favorite vegetables, herbs, and spices. Enjoy these delicious, heart-healthy, plant-based meals as part of a balanced, nutritious meal plan.

Days 35-37
Low-salt desserts and snacks
The Sprint Count Calories Cookbook for Fldglings believes that enjoying desserts and snacks while reducing salt levels can be part of a healthy lifestyle. On days 35-37, we'll introduce you to a selection of delicious desserts and treats that focus on salt intake without compromising

taste. These recipes will satisfy your sweet tooth while controlling your overall sodium intake. Explore these delicious, low-sodium options.

Day 35
New Natural product Serving of mixed greens with Mint-Lime Dressing
Make a revived natural product serving of mixed greens by combining an assortment of your favorite new natural products such as berries, melons, grapes, and citrus fragments. Get ready with a light dressing utilizing naturally crushed lime juice, a touch of nectar or maple syrup, and chopped new mint clears out. Hurl the natural product within the dressing and chill for some time recently. This straightforward and dynamic dessert is actually moo in sodium and bursting with characteristic sweetness.

Day 36
Dull Chocolate-Dipped Strawberries
Plunge new strawberries into softened dim chocolate, which is actually lower in sodium than drain chocolate. Permit the chocolate to set

some time recently getting a charge out of this delicious and antioxidant-rich treat. Keep in mind to select dim chocolate with a tall rate of cocoa for the greatest well-being benefits.

Day 37

Yogurt Parfait with Berries and Granola

Layer low-sodium Greek yogurt, new berries, and a sprinkle of hand-crafted granola in a glass or bowl. Rehash layers until the craved sum is come to. The combination of velvety yogurt, succulent berries, and crunchy granola gives a delightful and wholesome treat.

These reduced-sodium sweets and treats offer an extent of flavors and surfaces while keeping your sodium admissions in check. By utilizing actually low-sodium fixings and negligible or no included salt, you'll still enjoy delightful desserts without compromising your well-being objectives. Feel free to alter the formulas by consolidating your favorite natural products, nuts, or other flavorings to personalize your manifestations. Appreciate these delightful treats guilt-free of a well-balanced and careful eating arrangement.

Chapter 6

Dinner Arranging Methodologies for Fledglings

Setting out on a trip towards more advantageous eating propensities can be overpowering, particularly for apprentices. Supper arranging, in any case, gives a viable and viable arrangement. In this chapter, we'll investigate different dinner arranging procedures particularly custom-made for fledglings. By actualizing these methodologies, perusers of the "Sprint Check Calories Cookbook for Juveniles" can explore their way through the world of dinner arranging with certainty and ease.

Set clear objectives

Sometime recently you begin arranging your suppers, it's critical to set clear goals. Decide what you need to attain through your dinner arrangement. Whether it's weight misfortune, made strides in nourishment, or basically a more organized approach to dinners, having particular objectives will direct your arranging preparation and keep you persuaded.

Survey your dietary needs

Understanding your wholesome needs is key to making an effective meal arrangement. Consider any dietary limitations, hypersensitivities, or individual inclinations you will have. Additionally, evaluate your caloric prerequisites and supplement objectives to guarantee your dinners adjust along with your personal needs. Counseling with healthcare proficient or an enlisted dietitian can give profitable experiences in this regard.

Begin with a week-by-week arrangement

For tenderfoots, beginning with a week-after-week feast arrangement may be a sensible approach. Select a particular day of the week to sit down and arrange your meals for the up and coming week. Take into consideration your plan, including work, school, and other commitments, to decide the number of dinners you wish to arrange. Start with arranging breakfast, lunch, supper, and snacks for each day, guaranteeing they are well-balanced and meet your dietary objectives.

Utilize formula assets

Use the control of formula assets to make your feast arranging preparation simpler. The "Sprint Check Calories Cookbook for Juveniles" is an amazing beginning point, giving an assortment of beginner-friendly recipes. Investigate online formula websites, cookbooks, and indeed portable applications committed to supper arranging and formula recommendations. Explore formulas that adjust together with your dietary objectives and fit your cooking aptitudes and accessible fixings.

Clump cooking and remains

Make use of clump cooking to spare time and exertion. Plan bigger amounts of certain dishes, such as soups, stews, or simmered vegetables, that can be put away and utilized for numerous dinners all through the week. Scraps can be repurposed inventively, such as turning broiled chicken into a salad or using cooked grains in a stir-fry. By joining bunch cooking and scraps into your meal arrangement, you decrease the requirement for day-by-day extensive meal arrangement.

Make a shopping list

Once you have got your supper arranged, make a comprehensive shopping list based on the fixings required for your arranged meals. Having a shopping list ensures you simply purchase what you wish, lessening nourishment squander and superfluous costs. Adhere to your list when at the basic need store and consider shopping in bulk for non-perishable things to spare cash.

Prep in progress

To streamline your meal preparation process, consider prepping certain fixings in development. Wash and chop vegetables, marinate proteins, or pre-cook grains and vegetables ahead of time. These pre-prepared fixings can be put away in the fridge or cooler, prepared to be joined into your dinners all through the week. Prepping in development spares time and makes cooking more proficient.

Conclusion

Meal planning is a valuable skill that allows beginners to take control of their diet and eating habits. By setting clear goals, assessing nutritional needs, starting a weekly plan, leveraging recipe resources, incorporating batch cooking and leftovers, creating a grocery list, and prepping ahead of time, even a novice can make a meal. You can lay a solid foundation for a successful plan. Combining these strategies with the instructions and recipes in the Sprint Count Calories Cookbook for Chicks creates a seamless and enjoyable path to healthier eating.

Benefits of Solid Dinners

In today's fast-paced world, time and convenience make it easy to fall into the trap of unhealthy eating habits. But a solid dinner prep, also known as meal prep, is very important for anyone looking to improve their health and nutrition. This chapter explores the many benefits of preparing a healthy dinner and how it relates to readers of the Sprint Count Calories Cookbook for Chicks.

Time-saving convenience

One of the main benefits of preparing a solid dinner is that it saves you time. Taking a few hours on your chosen day to plan, prepare, and distribute your meals for the week can save you a lot of time and effort in the long run. Instant food saves you the daily hassle of deciding what to eat and cooking from scratch every day, especially if you don't have time.

Portion control and calorie control

Diet control and calorie management can be a daunting task for those just beginning their health and fitness journey. But a solid dinner prep can be an effective solution. By planning and preparing your meals in advance, you can better control portion sizes and ensure that your meals meet your desired calorie intake. This approach allows you to make conscious choices about the foods you eat and effectively reach your nutritional goals.

Nutritional balance

Maintaining a balanced diet is essential for overall health, but can be difficult without proper planning. By preparing a solid soup, you can create a balanced diet that contains all the essential nutrients your body needs. A balanced diet can be ensured through careful selection of a variety of ingredients, including lean proteins, whole grains, fruits, vegetables, and healthy fats. This approach improves overall health, boosts energy levels, and helps with weight management.

Improved dietary compliance

Sticking to a new diet or healthy eating plan can be difficult, especially when faced with tempting and unhealthy foods. However, preparing a solid dinner is a powerful tool for promoting dietary adherence. Having prepackaged, nutritious meals on hand reduces the chances of indulging in unhealthy cravings and resorting to fast and processed foods. Having healthy choices at hand makes it easier to stay on track and resist temptation.

Cost-effective and budget-friendly

Opposite to well-known conviction, strong dinner prep can really be cost-effective and budget-friendly. Once you plan your suppers in progress, you'll make a shopping list based on your formulas, guaranteeing you merely buy the vital fixings. By buying in bulk and utilizing remains productively, you'll be able to spare cash on goods and decrease nourishment squandering. Moreover, prepping your suppers can be more reasonable than feasting out or buying pre-packaged comfort nourishments.

Conclusion

Strong dinner prep offers various benefits to people looking to progress their well-being, oversee their calorie admissions, and keep up an adjusted eat-less. By grasping this hone, perusers of the "Sprint Tally Calories Cookbook for Juveniles" can saddle the control of supper prepping to streamline their travel towards more advantageous eating propensities. With time-saving comfort, parcel control, wholesome adjustment, improved adherence, and cost-effectiveness, strong dinner prep gets to be a priceless apparatus for accomplishing long-term victory in solid eating.

Planning Suppers in Progress

Tips and Procedures

Planning dinners in development, moreover known as feast prepping, could be a game-changing methodology for people looking for spare time, keeping up a sound count of calories, and remaining organized in their culinary endeavors. In this chapter, we'll explore valuable tips and procedures to offer assistance to readers of the "Sprint Check Calories Cookbook for Juveniles" in the art of planning suppers in development, making their cooking encounter more proficient, pleasant, and stress-free.

Arrange your dinners

Begin by arranging your suppers for the week. Consider your dietary objectives, preferences, and the number of dinners you would like to plan. See-through recipes, including those given within the cookbook, and select dishes that adjust together with your dietary needs and culinary abilities. Point for an adjustment of proteins, carbohydrates, and vegetables in each dinner to guarantee a well-rounded and fulfilling slim down.

Make a comprehensive shopping list

Once you have got your dinner arranged, make a shopping list that incorporates all the fixings required for your formulas. Take stock of your pantry, fridge, and cooler to maintain a strategic distance from superfluous buys and nourishment squandering. Organize your shopping list by areas of delivery, proteins, washroom things, etc. to form basic need shopping more productive and guarantee you do not disregard any fundamental fixings.

Choose an appropriate storage container
Invest in a collection of high-quality, airtight storage containers that can be frozen and microwaved. Choose from a variety of sizes to suit different portion sizes and meal types. Glass containers are popular because they are durable, easy to clean, and do not retain odors or stains. With the right storage containers, you can keep your cooked meals fresh, retain their flavor, and easily reheat them when needed.

Batch cooking and portioning

Batch cooking is a time-saving technique for preparing large batches of certain dishes or ingredients that can be used in multiple meals. For example, you can roast a whole chicken, grill a chicken breast, or cook quinoa in a large pot. Then divide the cooked ingredients into individual portions and store them in the refrigerator or freezer for later use. This allows you to mix and match ingredients to create a variety of meals throughout the week.

Prepare ingredients in advance
Preparing ingredients ahead of time streamlines the meal preparation process. Wash and chop vegetables, fruits, and herbs and store them in airtight containers or reusable bags. This makes it easier and faster to put together a meal when you're ready to cook. Plus, marinate proteins, prepare homemade sauces and dressings, and pre-cook grains and legumes. The ready availability of ready-made ingredients reduces cooking time and simplifies meal composition.

Use freezer-safe recipes

Get the most out of your freezer by preparing freezer-safe meals. These may be fully-cooked dishes or partially prepared-components that can be assembled and cooked later. Casseroles, soups, stews, and sauces are great for freezing. Divide it into individual pieces and label them with your name and date so you can keep track of them. Freezer-safe meals are great for busy days or when you need a quick, nutritious option.

Ensuring proper food safety

When preparing food, it is important to prioritize food safety. Always allow cooked food to cool to room temperature before refrigerating or freezing to prevent bacterial growth. Follow proper storage guidelines and date-label containers to track freshness. If reheating a cooked meal, make sure it reaches a safe internal temperature to eliminate bacteria.

Rotate and vary your diet

To prevent fatigue while eating and ensure a balanced diet, rotate and vary your meals throughout the week. Mix and match proteins, grains, and veggies for cooked meals to add interest. Incorporate different flavors, spices, and recipes to add variety to your diet. This not only prevents boredom but also ensures that you are getting a variety of nutrients.

Hone effective assembly-line cooking

When it's time to collect and parcel your prepared suppers, receive an effective assembly-line approach. Set up your workspace with all the fundamental fixings, holders, and utensils. Work in an orderly way, gathering each feast one by one. This spares time and minimizes clean-up.

Name and organize your dinners

To remain organized, name each holder with the title of the dish and the date it was arranged. This makes a difference if you keep track of the freshness of your dinners and guarantees you expend them inside a secure time outline.

Organize your prepared dinners in the fridge or cooler, orchestrating them in a way that permits simple get-to and permeability.

Consider theme-based supper prepping

To include energy in your feast prep schedule, consider theme-based supper prepping. Select a cooking or flavor profile and arrange your suppers around it. For illustration, you may have a Mexican-themed week with dishes like tacos, burrito bowls, and enchiladas. This approach includes assortment and keeps your taste buds fulfilled.

Grasp the flexibility of remains

Remains can be a supper prepper's best companion. Do not be anxious to repurpose and change your remains into unused and energizing dishes. Extra fricasseed chicken can be utilized in servings of mixed greens, sandwiches, stir-fries, and more. Get imaginative and explore distinctive combinations to diminish squandering and make the most out of your prepared dinners.

Conclusion

Planning dinners in advance through meal prepping could be a viable and efficient approach to keeping up a sound count of calories and sparing time in the kitchen. By taking after the tips and techniques outlined in this chapter, perusers of the "Sprint Check Calories Cookbook for Juveniles" can end up capable of dinner prepping, making their cooking involvement more streamlined and agreeable. With appropriate arranging, portioning, fixing planning, and capacity, planning dinners in progress gets to be an important apparatus in keeping up a nutritious and well-balanced slim down, indeed for those with active plans.

Chapter 7

Appropriate Capacity and Solidifying Procedures

Legitimate capacity and solidifying procedures are basic aptitudes for people locked in in feast prepping and looking to preserve the freshness and quality of their arranged meals. In this chapter, we'll dig into the finest homes for putting away prepared suppers, fixings, and remains to maximize their rack life and protect their flavors and surfaces. By taking after these methods, users of the "Sprint Number Calories Cookbook for Juveniles' can ensure that their dinners are secure, delicious, and prepared to appreciate when required.

Select the proper holders

Selecting the correct capacity holders is crucial for keeping up the judgment of your prepared dinners. Pick holders that are sealed shut, leak-proof, and freezer-safe. Glass holders are a favored choice as they don't hold odors or stains and are microwave-safe. On the off chance that utilizing plastic holders, guarantee they are labeled as microwave-safe and BPA-free. Contribute totally different sizes to suit different parcel sizes and guarantee a cozy fit.

Cool cooked dinners some-time recently putting away

Some-time recently putting away cooked dinners, permit them to cool to room temperature. Hot nourishment can raise the temperature inside the fridge or cooler, compromising the security and quality of other put-away things. Partition bigger parcels into personal servings to encourage faster cooling. Once cooled, cover the holders firmly and put them in the refrigerator or cooler promptly.

Name holders with dates and substance

Naming your capacity holders with the dates and substance is basic for remaining organized and keeping track of freshness. Utilize detachable names or freezer-safe markers to show the date the supper was arranged or put away. Moreover, name the substance or name of the dish to effectively identify the put-away things. This makes a difference, anticipates disarray, and permits you to expend meals within a secure time period.

Utilize legitimate portioning and bundling strategies

When portioning meals for capacity, consider the serving sizes and your planning utilization. Partition bigger dishes into personal parcels to guarantee simple grab-and-go options. Package each parcel in partitioned holders to maintain a strategic distance from having to defrost and refreeze bigger parcels over and over. This permits you to thaw only what you would, like decreasing squandering and keeping up the quality of the remaining parcels.

Take after prescribed capacity times
Distinctive sorts of nourishment have changed suggested capacity times. It's vital to follow these rules to guarantee nourishment, security, and quality. Cooked meats, poultry, and angle can by and large be put away in the fridge for up to four days, whereas cooked grains, vegetables, and sauces can final for three to five days. In case you're not arranging to devour the dinners inside the prescribed time allotment, consider solidifying them for a longer capacity.

Utilize appropriate solidifying methods
Solidifying is a fabulous strategy for expanding the rack life of your prepared dinners. Be that as it may, it's critical to take after legitimate solidifying procedures to protect flavor and surface. Permit hot nourishments to cool totally some-time recently solidifying to maintain a strategic distance from ice gem arrangement and dampness buildup. For ideal comes about, bundle your suppers firmly, taking off negligible discuss space interior the holders to anticipate

cooler burn. Consider utilizing vacuum-sealed packs or evacuating abundance from zip-top packs for made strides in conservation.

Name and date cooler things

Legitimately name and date your cooler things to keep track of their capacity time. Utilize freezer-safe names or markers to demonstrate the title of the dish and the date it was solidified. This hone makes a difference you effectively recognize and turn your cooler things, guaranteeing you expend the most seasoned dinners, to begin with.

Defrost and warm with care

When it's time to appreciate your prepared suppers, defrost them and warm them with care. To defrost solidified suppers, exchange them from the cooler to the fridge a day in development. You'll moreover utilize the defrost work of the microwave. Dodge defrosting at room temperature as this may empower bacterial development. When warming, take after the prescribed rules for each particular supper. Guarantee that warmed suppers reaches a secure inner temperature to dispense with any potential microscopic organisms. Mix and pivot the nourishment amid warming to guarantee indeed warming and protect the surface.

Consider the appropriateness of certain fixings for solidifying

Whereas numerous fixings can be effectively solidified, a few may not hold their quality or surface after defrosting. Fixings with tall water substances, such as lettuce, cucumbers, and fragile herbs, don't solidify well. So also, dishes with velvety or mayonnaise-based sauces may be partitioned when defrosted. Consider these variables when arranging your prepared suppers to guarantee the most excellent comes about.

Appropriately store and name scraps

Scraps from your naturally cooked suppers too require appropriate capacity and labeling. Put them in airtight containers and refrigerate them instantly. Name the holder with the date and substance to track freshness. Devour remaining dinners inside the recommended capacity time, regularly 3-4 days, to preserve their quality and security.

Refining the principle of "first in, first out".
To play down nourishment squander and guarantee freshness, hone the "primary in, to begin without" rule. Orchestrate your put-away dinners and fixings within the fridge and cooler in a way that permits simple get to the most seasoned things. This way, you prioritize expanding the dinners that have been put away the longest some-time recently moving on to more up-to-date increments.

Pay consideration to the cooler organization
Keep up an organized cooler by gathering comparative things together. Keep raw meat and fish isolated from other nourishments to maintain a strategic distance from cross-contamination. Consider utilizing cooler wicker containers or dividers to form assigned segments

for diverse sorts of suppers or fixings. Routinely clean and defrost your cooler to preserve ideal solidifying conditions and anticipate ice buildup.

Conclusion

Appropriate capacity and solidifying methods are crucial for keeping up the quality, flavor, and security of your prepared dinners, fixings, and scraps. By taking after the rules sketched out in this chapter, perusers of the "Sprint Tally Calories Cookbook for Juveniles" can certainly store and solidify their suppers with ease. Following suggested capacity times, utilizing suitable holders, labeling and dating things, and practicing proper thawing and warming strategies will guarantee that your prepped meals remain delightful, helpful, and secure for utilization. With these procedures, you'll make the foremost of your feast-prepping endeavors and appreciate wholesome and flavorful suppers at whatever point you want.

Chapter 8

Making Healthy Choices When Eating Out

Eating out can be a delightful experience, offering a break from cooking and a chance to explore different cuisines. However, it can also present challenges when trying to maintain a healthy diet. In this chapter, we will explore strategies and tips for making smart and nutritious choices when dining out. By applying these techniques, readers of the "Sprint Count Calories Cookbook for Fledglings" can navigate restaurant menus with confidence and enjoy meals that align with their health goals.

Research restaurants in advance

Before heading out, look for nearby restaurants. Look for establishments that offer healthier menu options, such as those with vegetarian or vegan choices, farm-to-table concepts, or menus that prioritize fresh, locally sourced ingredients. Reading online reviews and checking out the restaurant's website can give you insights into it's menu offerings and overall commitment to healthy dining.

Plan ahead

If possible, review the menu of the chosen restaurant ahead of time. Look for dishes that are rich in lean proteins, whole grains, and vegetables. Avoid menu items that are fried, heavily processed, or loaded with added sugars and unhealthy fats. By planning your order in advance, you're less likely to make impulsive choices based on cravings or hunger.

Practice portion control

The portions in restaurants are often more than what is needed for a single meal. To avoid overeating, either share the main course with the person at the table next to you or ask the waiter to combine half the meals before serving. Alternatively, order an appetizer or a side dish as your main course. If you do have a large portion, practice mindful eating by listening to your body's cues and stopping when you feel satisfied, rather than finishing everything on your plate.

Choose healthier cooking methods

Opt for dishes that are prepared using healthier cooking methods, such as grilling, baking, steaming, or broiling, rather than fried or deep-fried options. These methods typically use less oil and retain more nutrients in the food. If a dish you desire is typically fried, ask the server if it can be prepared using a healthier cooking technique.

Pay attention to ingredients and preparation

Be mindful of the ingredients used in the dishes you're considering. Look for options that incorporate whole foods, fresh produce, and lean proteins. Avoid dishes that are heavily processed, loaded with preservatives, or high in sodium. Additionally, ask the server about the preparation methods, such as whether the dish is cooked with excessive oils or butter. Request modifications or substitutions to make the dish healthier, such as dressing or sauce on the side or opting for whole-grain bread or pasta.

Center on natural products and vegetables

When requesting, prioritize dishes that incorporate a liberal parcel of natural products and vegetables. These are nutrient-dense and give fundamental vitamins, minerals, and fiber. Select servings of mixed greens, vegetable sides, or dishes that join an assortment of colorful delivery. You'll be able to inquire about additional vegetables in your dishes or ask for a side of steamed vegetables.

Intellect your refreshments

Refreshments can include a parcel of calories and sugar to eat less. Unsweetened tea, or shimmering water rather than sugary soft drinks, sweetened cocktails, or high-calorie refreshments. On the off chance that you lean toward liquor, select lighter alternatives like wine or a light brew, and constrain your admissions.

Be careful of condiments and dressings

Condiments and dressings can include an abundance of calories, undesirable fats, and sodium in your meal. Ask for dressings and sauces on the side, so you'll control the sum you utilize. Consider more advantageous choices like olive oil and vinegar or take lighter dressings. Utilize condiments sparingly or select lower-sodium alternatives when accessible.

Be emphatic when requesting

Do not be anxious to inquire questions or make uncommon demands when making your arrangements. Eateries are regularly willing to suit dietary inclinations or alterations. For example, you'll request barbecued or steamed alternatives rather than fricasseed, ask for sauces or dressings on the side, or substitute high-calorie sides with more beneficial options like steamed vegetables or a side serving of mixed greens. Keep in mind, it's your feast, and the eatery needs you to have a positive eating involvement.

Hone careful eating

Eating out should be an agreeable encounter, but it's critical to remain careful of your nourishment choices and eating propensities. Moderate down and savor each nibble, paying consideration to flavors and surfaces. Tune in to your body's starvation and satiety signals and halt eating after you feel full. Maintain a strategic distance from diversions like phones or tv screens, as they can lead to thoughtless eating. Engage in discussions along with your eating companions and center on the social angle of eating.

Choose healthier side dishes

Many restaurant meals come with side dishes that have a significant impact on the nutritional value of the overall meal. Choose healthier side dishes, such as steamed vegetables, side salads with dressings, and side dishes with whole grains like quinoa or brown rice. If you don't have a side to match your meal, ask if a substitute side can be made or if the side can be ordered separately.

Make generous choices and practice moderation

It's okay to indulge once in a while and enjoy your favorite snacks and meals while you eat. But try to keep moderation and balance. If you want to eat desserts or high-calorie dishes, consider sharing them with a dining companion or choosing smaller dishes. You can even enjoy a healthier main course and take a few of your favorite treats to use later.

Summary

Eating out doesn't have to get in the way of a healthy diet. By following the strategies and tips outlined in these chapters, readers of "The Sprint Count Calories Cookbook for Fledglings" can help make informed and nutritious choices when dining out. From pre-planning and researching options to practicing portion control, choosing healthier ingredients, and making conscious choices in your choices, choose restaurant menus with confidence and eat delicious food that supports your health and well-being. Remember, making healthy choices when eating out means finding balance and enjoying the experience while nourishing your body with healthy food.